84 Organic Solutions to Diarrhea and Stomach Problems:

Juice and Meal Recipes to Help You Recover Fast

By

Joe Correa CSN

COPYRIGHT

ACKNOWLEDGEMENTS

This book is dedicated to my friends and family that have had mild or serious illnesses so that you may find a solution and make the necessary changes in your life.

84 Organic Solutions to Diarrhea and Stomach Problems:

Juice and Meal Recipes to Help You Recover Fast

By

Joe Correa CSN

CONTENTS

ABOUT THE AUTHOR

After years of Research, I honestly believe in the positive effects that proper nutrition can have over the body and mind. My knowledge and experience has helped me live healthier throughout the years and which I have shared with family and friends. The more you know about eating and drinking healthier, the sooner you will want to change your life and eating habits.

Nutrition is a key part in the process of being healthy and living longer so get started today. The first step is the most important and the most significant.

INTRODUCTION

84 Organic Solutions to Diarrhea and Stomach Problems: Juice and Meal Recipes to Help You Recover Fast

By Joe Correa CSN

Frequent loose and watery stools caused by an increased secretion of fluid into the intestine and reduced absorption of fluid from the intestine is known as diarrhea. This condition usually lasts for just a couple of days and goes away on its own. In some more severe cases, diarrhea can last up to 3-4 weeks and sometimes even develop into a chronic disease.

Diarrhea is a medical condition that can affect most of the population, regardless of age or sex. Most adults in the United States have diarrhea at least once a year. Children, on the other hand, tend to suffer from diarrhea more often, on average twice per year.

Diarrhea can be caused by different factors. The most common include:

- Contaminated food or water

- Different viruses

- Some parasites found in food or water

- Various medicines

- Problems with digestion of certain foods and food intolerances (like lactose intolerance)

- Diseases of the digestive tract

- Irritable bowel syndrome

Diarrhea is often followed by common and recognizable symptoms like sharp pain and cramps in the abdomen, an urgent and uncontrollable need to use the bathroom, and liquid stools. Naturally, this condition can cause dehydration which can be quite dangerous, especially for newborns and older people. In this case, urgent medical attention is needed.

When it comes to treatment, in most cases, diarrhea goes away on its own. However, rehydration is extremely important in order to replace lost fluids in the body. People suffering from diarrhea are often advised to drink plenty of fruit and vegetable juices, sodas without caffeine, and broths. In more serious cases, oral rehydration solutions are often prescribed.

This book contains some fantastic juice recipes that were carefully chosen to help eliminate diarrhea and rehydrate the entire body. These juices are based on fresh fruits and vegetables that have the ability to clean the entire digestive tract and help your body heal within a couple of days. Furthermore, these juices take only a couple of minutes to prepare which means you can enjoy them all day long.

Give these juices a try and see which ones you like the most!

COMMITMENT

In order to improve my condition, I *(your name)*, commit to eating more of these foods on a daily basis and to exercise at least 30 minutes daily:

- Berries (especially blueberries), peaches, cherries, apples, apricots, oranges, lemon juice, grapefruit, tangerines, mandarins, pears, etc.
- Broccoli, spinach, collard greens, sweet potatoes, avocado, artichoke, baby corn, carrots, celery, cauliflower, onions, etc.
- Whole grains, steel-cut oats, oatmeal, quinoa, barley, etc.
- Black beans, red bean beans, garbanzo beans, lentils, etc.
- Nuts and seeds including: walnuts, cashews, flaxseeds, sesame seeds, etc.
- Fish
- 8 – 10 glasses of water

Sign here

X_____

84 ORGANIC SOLUTIONS TO DIARRHEA AND STOMACH PROBLEMS

JUICES

1.   **Banana Blueberry Juice**

Ingredients:

2 large bananas, peeled

1 cup blueberries, fresh

1 medium-sized radish, sliced

1 tbsp fresh mint, chopped

1 cup cauliflower, chopped

¼ cup water

Preparation:

Peel the bananas and cut into thin slices. Set aside.

Wash the blueberries under cold running water. Drain and set aside.

Wash the radish and trim off the green parts. Cut into small pieces and set aside.

Trim off the outer leaves of cauliflower. Wash it and cut into small pieces. Reserve the rest in the refrigerator.

Now, combine bananas, blueberries, radish, cauliflower and mint in a juicer. Process until juiced.

Transfer to serving glasses and stir in the coconut water.

Add some ice and serve.

Nutritional information per serving: Kcal: 232, Protein: 5.2g, Carbs: 98.9g, Fats: 1.7g

2.   Artichoke Brussels Sprout Juice

Ingredients:

1 large artichoke, chopped

1 cup Brussels sprouts, chopped

1 cup mustard greens, chopped

1 medium-sized Red Delicious apple, peeled and cored

½ tsp cinnamon, freshly ground

½ cup coconut water, unsweetened

1 tsp honey

Preparation:

Trim off the outer leave of the artichoke using a sharp knife. Rinse well and cut into small pieces. Set aside.

Rinse the Brussels sprouts and trim off the outer layers. Chop into small pieces and set aside.

Place the mustard greens in a large colander and rinse under running water. Torn into small pieces and set aside.

Wash the apple and remove the core. Cut into bite-sized pieces and set aside.

Now, place artichoke, Brussels sprouts, mustard greens, and apple in a juicer. Process until juiced.

Transfer to serving glasses and stir in the cinnamon, coconut water, and honey.

Add some ice and serve immediately.

Nutritional information per serving: Kcal: 195, Protein: 13.7g, Carbs: 63.4g, Fats: 1.3g

3.   Beet Juice

Ingredients:

1 cup beets, trimmed

1 cup beet greens, chopped

1 cup cauliflower, chopped

1 cup parsnips, chopped

2 tbsp fresh mint, finely chopped

Preparation:

Wash the beets and trim off the green parts. Cut into small pieces. Chop the greens and set aside.

Wash the parsnips and cut into thick slices. Set aside.

Trim off the outer leaves of a cauliflower. Wash it and chop into small pieces. Set aside.

Now, combine beets, beet greens, cauliflower, and parsnips in a juicer. Process until juiced.

Transfer to serving glasses and refrigerate for 10 minutes. Garnish with fresh mint before serving.

Nutritional information per serving: Kcal: 167, Protein: 9.8g, Carbs: 52.8g, Fats: 1.6g

4.   Honeycrisp Chia Juice

Ingredients:

1 small Honeycrisp apple, cored

1 cup cucumber, sliced

½ red bell pepper, seeded

½ yellow bell pepper, seeded

3 tbsp chia seeds

Preparation:

Peel the cucumber and cut into thin slices. Fill the measuring cup and reserve the rest in the refrigerator.

Rinse peppers and cut in half. Remove the seeds and chop one-half into small pieces. Place in a bowl. Reserve the rest in the refrigerator.

Wash the apple and remove the core. Cut into bite-sized pieces and set aside.

Now, combine cucumber, bell peppers, and apple in a juicer. Transfer to serving glasses and stir in the chia seeds.

Refrigerate for 15 minutes before serving.

Enjoy!

Nutritional information per serving: Kcal: 136, Protein: 4.3g, Carbs: 31.2g, Fats: 6.1g

5.   Banana Apricot Juice

Ingredients:

1 large banana, chunked

1 large apricot, pitted

1 cup cauliflower florets, chopped

1 cup broccoli, chopped

Preparation:

Peel the banana and cut into small chunks. Set aside.

Wash the apricot and cut in half. Remove the pit and cut into small pieces. Set aside.

Rinse the cauliflower florets under running water using a colander. Drain and set aside.

Place the broccoli in a colander and wash under cold running water. Chop into small pieces and set aside.

Combine banana, apricot, grapefruit, and broccoli in a juicer. Transfer to serving glasses and refrigerate for 30 minutes before serving.

Nutritional information per serving: Kcal: 229, Protein: 6.5g, Carbs: 67.2g, Fats: 1.3g

6.   Apple Carrot Juice

Ingredients:

1 large Golden Delicious apple, peeled and cored

1 large carrot, sliced

½ cup of butternut squash, chopped

1 tbsp of fresh mint, finely chopped

1 large banana, sliced

¼ tsp ginger, ground

Preparation:

Wash the apple and remove the core. Cut into bite-sized pieces and set aside.

Wash the carrot and cut into small slices. Set aside.

Peel the butternut squash and remove the seeds using a spoon. Cut into small cubes and reserve the rest of the squash for some other recipe. Wrap in a plastic foil and refrigerate.

Peel the banana and cut into thin slices. Set aside.

Now, combine apple carrot, butternut squash, and banana in a juicer. Process until juiced.

Transfer to serving glasses and stir in the mint for some extra taste.

Add some ice and serve.

Nutritional information per serving: Kcal: 372, Protein: 5.5g, Carbs: 73.4g, Fats: 1.4g

7. Leek Brussels Sprout Juice

Ingredients:

2 whole leeks, chopped

1 cup of Brussels sprouts, chopped

1 cup of parsley, chopped

A handful of spinach, chopped

½ cup of water

Preparation:

Wash the leeks and chop into small pieces. Set aside.

Wash the Brussels sprouts and trim off the outer leaves. Cut in half and set aside.

Wash the parsley in a colander under cold running water and set aside.

Wash the spinach thoroughly and set aside.

Combine leeks, Brussels sprouts, parsley, and spinach in a juicer. Transfer to serving glasses and stir in the water.

Refrigerate for 10 minutes before serving.

Nutritional information per serving: Kcal: 120, Protein: 6.4g, Carbs: 46.2g, Fats: 1.8g

8.   Cabbage Carrot Juice

Ingredients:

2 cups of green cabbage, shredded

1 cup of carrots, chopped

2 small Granny Smith's apples, core

1 large banana, peeled

1 tbsp of honey, raw

Preparation:

Wash the cabbage thoroughly and roughly chop it using hands. Set aside.

Wash the carrots and cut into small pieces. Set aside.

Peel the apples and cut in half. Remove the core and cut into bite-sized pieces. Set aside.

Peel the banana and cut into thin slices. Set aside.

Now, combine cabbage, carrots, apples, and banana in a juicer. Process until juiced.

Transfer to serving glasses and stir in the honey.

Add some ice cubes and serve immediately.

Nutritional information per serving: Kcal: 219, Protein: 6.9g, Carbs: 69g, Fats: 1.5g

9. Maple Peach Juice

Ingredients:

1 large peach, peeled

1 cup parsnip, sliced

½ cup strawberries, chopped

3 cups lettuce, torn

1 tsp maple syrup

Preparation:

Rinse the peach and cut in half. Remove the pit and cut into bite-sized pieces. Set aside.

Wash and peel the parsnips. Cut into thick slices and set aside.

Rinse the strawberries and remove the stems. Cut into halves and set aside.

Rinse the lettuce thoroughly using a colander. Torn into small pieces and set aside.

Now, combine peach, parsnips, strawberries, and lettuce in a juicer. Process until juiced. Transfer to serving glasses and stir in the maple syrup.

Add some ice and serve immediately.

Nutritional information per serving: Kcal: 186, Protein: 5.4g, Carbs: 63.7g, Fats: 1.1g

10.   Mango Banana Juice

Ingredients:

1 large mango

1 large banana, peeled

1 large guava, peeled

¼ cup coconut water

Preparation:

Peel the mango and cut into small chunks. Set aside.

Peel the banana and cut into thin slices. Set aside.

Wash the guava and cut into chunks. If you are using large fruit, reserve the rest for some other recipe in a refrigerator. Set aside.

Now, combine mango, banana, and guava in a juicer. Transfer to serving glasses and stir in the coconut water.

Add few ice cubes and serve immediately.

Enjoy!

Nutritional information per serving: Kcal: 295, Protein: 4.4g, Carbs: 88.9g, Fats: 1.8g

11.   Cabbage Apple Juice

Ingredients:

1 cup of green cabbage, chopped

1 large Fuji apple, cored

1 cup of pumpkin, seeded and peeled

1 large banana, peeled

¼ tsp ginger powder

Preparation:

Rinse the cabbage thoroughly using a colander. Chop into small pieces and set aside.

Wash the apple and remove the core. Cut into bite-sized pieces and set aside.

Peel the pumpkin and cut in half. Scoop out the seeds using a spoon. Cut one large wedge and peel it. Cut into small chunks and set aside.

Peel the banana and cut into thin slices. Set aside.

Now, combine cabbage, apple, pumpkin, and banana in a juicer. Transfer to serving glasses and add few ice cubes.

Refrigerate for 10-15 minutes before serving.

Nutritional information per serving: Kcal: 228, Protein: 5.4g, Carbs: 69.3g, Fats: 1.5g

12.   Radish Mint Juice

Ingredients:

1 medium-sized radish, chopped

1 tbsp of fresh mint, chopped

1 cup of cantaloupe, diced

1 cup of beet greens, chopped

1 cup of cauliflower, chopped

Preparation:

Wash the radish and trim off the green parts. Cut into small chunks and set aside.

Soak the mint leaves in water. Let it stand for 2 minutes.

Trim off the outer leaves of cauliflower. Wash it and cut into small pieces. Reserve the rest in the refrigerator.

Cut the cantaloupe in half. Scoop out the seeds and flesh. Cut two wedges and peel them. Chop into chunks and set aside. Reserve the rest of the cantaloupe in a refrigerator.

Wash the beet greens and torn with hands. Set aside.

Now, combine cantaloupe, beet greens, radish, cauliflower and mint in a juicer. Process until juiced.

Transfer to serving glasses and add some ice before serving.

Nutritional information per serving: Kcal: 123, Protein: 8.1g, Carbs: 37.7g, Fats: 1.1g

13.   Grape Broccoli Juice

Ingredients:

½ cup of black grapes

1 cup broccoli, chopped

1 medium-sized pear, roughly chopped

1 cup of spinach, torn

1 small ginger root slice, peeled

Preparation:

Wash the pear and remove the core. Cut into small pieces and set aside.

Rinse the broccoli and cut into small pieces. Fill the measuring cup and reserve the rest in the refrigerator.

Wash the grapes in a colander under cold running water and set aside.

Wash the spinach thoroughly and torn with hands. Set aside.

Peel the ginger slice and set aside.

Combine pear, grapes, oranges, spinach, and ginger in a juicer and process until juiced.

Transfer to serving glasses and refrigerate for 15 minutes before serving.

Enjoy!

Nutritional information per serving: Kcal: 217, Protein: 6.2g, Carbs: 75.4g, Fats: 1.2g

14.   Spinach Coconut Juice

Ingredients:

2 cups fresh spinach

½ cup of coconut water, unsweetened

1 cup of broccoli, chopped

1 tbsp of honey, raw

A few mint leaves

Preparation:

Wash the broccoli and trim off the outer leaves. Set aside.

Rinse the spinach thoroughly under running water. Drain and torn with hands. Set aside.

Now, combine broccoli and spinach in a juicer. Process until juiced.

Transfer to serving glasses and stir in the honey and garnish with mint leaves.

Add some ice and serve immediately.

Nutritional information per serving: Kcal: 171, Protein: 14.8g, Carbs: 54.5g, Fats: 2.17g

15.   Watermelon Spinach Juice

Ingredients:

2 cups watermelon, roughly chopped

2 cups spinach, chopped

2 cups fresh strawberries, chopped

1 medium-sized banana, peeled

½ tsp of cinnamon, ground

1 tsp of honey, raw

Preparation:

Cut the watermelon in half. Cut two large wedges and peel. Cut into small chunks and remove the seeds. Fill the measuring cups and reserve the rest for later.

Rinse the spinach thoroughly and torn with hands. Set aside.

Rinse the strawberries under cold running water and remove the stems. Chop into small pieces and set aside.

Peel the banana and cut into small chunks. Set aside.

Now, combine strawberries, melon, spinach, and banana in a juicer. Process until juiced. Transfer to serving glasses and stir in the honey and cinnamon.

Refrigerate for 10 minutes before serving minutes.

Nutritional information per serving: Kcal: 349, Protein: 7.6g, Carbs: 104.9g, Fats: 3.2g

16.   Blueberry Coconut Juice

Ingredients:

2 cups strawberries, chopped

1 cup blueberries

½ cup coconut water, unsweetened

1 tsp agave nectar

Preparation:

Combine blueberries and strawberries in a colander and wash under cold running water. Set aside.

Peel the orange and divide into wedges. Use about half of the wedges and reserve the rest for some other juice.

Combine blueberries and strawberries in a juicer. Transfer to serving glasses and stir in the coconut water and agave nectar.

Add some ice or refrigerate before serving.

Nutritional information per serving: Kcal: 246, Protein: 4.7g, Carbs: 74.2g, Fats: 1.7g

17.   Sweet Apple Banana Juice

Ingredients:

2 large Granny Smith apples, cored and chopped

1 large banana, peeled

1 tsp of honey, raw

½ tsp of ginger, freshly ground

Preparation:

Wash the apples and remove the core. Chop into bite-sized pieces and set aside.

Peel the banana and cut into thin slices. Set aside.

Now, combine apples and banana in a juicer. Transfer to serving glasses and stir in the honey and ginger.

Refrigerate or add some ice and serve.

Enjoy!

Nutritional information per serving: Kcal: 299, Protein: 3.7g, Carbs: 88g, Fats: 1.1g

18.   Cucumber Fuji Juice

Ingredients:

3 large cucumbers, peeled

1 Fuji apple, peeled

1 tsp peppermint extract

1 tbsp fresh mint, chopped

Preparation:

Wash the cucumbers and cut into thick slices. Set aside.

Peel the apple and remove the core. Cut into bite-sized pieces and set aside.

Now, combine cucumber and apple in a juicer and process until juiced. Transfer to serving glasses and stir in the peppermint extract.

Add some ice cubes and serve immediately.

Nutritional information per serving: Kcal: 204, Protein: 7.7g, Carbs: 59g, Fats: 1.3g

19. Banana Raspberry Juice

Ingredients:

1 large banana, peeled

1 cup raspberries, fresh

1 cup butternut squash, chopped

½ cup coconut water

1 tsp honey

Preparation:

Peel the banana and cut into chunks. Set aside.

Wash the raspberries under cold running water. Drain and set aside.

Peel the butternut squash and remove the seeds using a spoon. Cut into small cubes and reserve the rest of the squash for some other recipe. Wrap in a plastic foil and refrigerate.

Now, combine banana, raspberries, and butternut squash in a juicer. Transfer to serving glasses and stir in the coconut water and honey.

Add some ice and serve immediately.

Enjoy!

Nutritional information per serving: Kcal: 197, Protein: 4.7g, Carbs: 68g, Fats: 1.3g

20. Kale Cranberry Juice

Ingredients:

1 cup fresh kale, torn

1 cup cranberries

1 small Honeycrisp apple, cored

¼ cup coconut water

Preparation:

Peel the kiwis and cut lengthwise in half. Set aside.

Rinse the kale thoroughly and into small pieces. Fill the measuring cup and set aside.

Wash the cranberries under cold running water. Drain and set aside.

Now, combine kale, cranberries, and apple in a juicer. Transfer to serving glasses and stir in the coconut water.

Add some ice and serve immediately.

Nutritional information per serving: Kcal: 153, Protein: 5.6g, Carbs: 48.4g, Fats: 1.8g

21.   Blackberry Banana Juice

Ingredients:

2 cups blackberries

1 large banana, peeled

2 cups spinach, chopped

2 cups beet greens, chopped

¼ cup water

Preparation:

Rinse the blackberries under cold running water. Drain and set aside.

Peel the banana and cut into chunks. Set aside.

Combine spinach and beet greens in a colander and wash thoroughly. Chop into small pieces and set aside.

Now, combine blackberries, banana, spinach, and beet greens in a juicer. Process until juiced.

Transfer to serving glasses and add some ice cubes before serving.

Enjoy!

Nutritional information per serving: Kcal: 183, Protein: 7.8g, Carbs: 63.1g, Fats: 1.2g

22.　　Blackberry Turnip Juice

Ingredients:

1 cup of plums, halved

1 cup of fresh blackberries

1 cup of turnip greens, chopped

½ tsp of ginger, ginger

½ cup of water

Preparation:

Rinse the blackberries under cold running water using a colander. Drain and set aside.

Rinse the turnip greens and torn into small pieces. Set aside.

Wash the plums and cut in half. Remove the pits and set aside.

Now, combine plums, blackberries, and turnip greens in a juicer and process until juiced.

Transfer to serving glasses and stir in the ginger and water.

Refrigerate for 5 minutes before serving.

Enjoy!

Nutritional information per serving: Kcal: 141, Protein: 4.2g, Carbs: 40.3g, Fats: 1.4g

23.   Radish Beet Juice

Ingredients:

2 cups radishes, chopped

1 cup of beet greens, torn

1 cup of watercress, chopped

1 tbsp of honey, raw

Preparation:

Wash the radishes and trim off the green parts. Cut into small pieces and set aside.

Place the beet greens and watercress in a large colander. Rinse under cold running water and torn into small pieces.

Now, combine radishes, beet greens, and watercress in a juicer and process until juiced.

Transfer to serving glasses and add some ice before serving.

Enjoy!

Nutritional information per serving: Kcal: 147, Protein: 5.3g, Carbs: 50g, Fats: 0.8g

24.   Peach Spinach Juice

Ingredients:

1 large peach, chopped

1 cup spinach, torn

2 large Red Delicious apples, peeled and cored

1 large carrot, sliced

¼ cup water

Preparation:

Wash the peach and cut in half. Remove the pit and chop into small pieces. Set aside.

Rinse the spinach thoroughly and torn with hands. Set aside.

Wash the apples and remove the core. Cut into thin slices and set aside.

Wash the carrot and cut into thick slices. Set aside.

Now, combine apples, peach, spinach, and carrot in a juicer and process until juiced.

Transfer to serving glasses and refrigerate for 10 minutes before serving.

Nutritional information per serving: Kcal: 297, Protein: 5.5g, Carbs: 87.5g, Fats: 1.5g

25.   Broccoli Coconut Juice

Ingredients:

2 cups raw broccoli, chopped

½ cup coconut water

1 cup fresh raspberries

2 large cucumbers, peeled

1 tbsp honey

Preparation:

Wash the raspberries under cold running water. Drain and set aside.

Wash the broccoli and cut into small pieces. Set aside.

Wash and peel the cucumbers. Cut into thick slices and set aside.

Combine broccoli, cucumber, and raspberries in a juicer and process until juiced.

Transfer to serving glasses and stir in the coconut water and honey.

Add some ice and serve.

Nutritional information per serving: Kcal: 192, Protein: 10.9g, Carbs: 56g, Fats: 2.2g

26. Leek Brussels Sprout Juice

Ingredients:

1 whole leek, chopped

1 cup of Brussels sprouts, chopped

1 large green apple, peeled and seeds removed

2 cups of mustard greens, chopped

1 medium-sized zucchini, peeled

1 cup of parsnip, sliced

Preparation:

Wash the leek and cut into small pieces. Set aside.

Wash the Brussels sprouts and trim off the outer leaves. Set aside.

Wash the apple and remove the core. Cut into bite-sized pieces and set aside.

Wash the mustard greens and torn with hands. Set aside.

Wash the zucchini and cut in half. Scoop out the seeds using a spoon. Cut into small chunks and set aside.

Wash the parsnips and cut into thick slices. Set aside.

Now, combine leek, Brussels sprouts, apple, mustard greens, zucchini and parsnips in a juicer.

Transfer to serving glasses and refrigerate for 5 minutes before serving.

Nutritional information per serving: Kcal: 284, Protein: 12.3g, Carbs: 83.7g, Fats: 2.4g

27.   Cabbage Apple Juice

Ingredients:

1 cup of purple cabbage, torn

1 Granny Smith's apple, cored

1 cup of red leaf lettuce, torn

1 cup of papaya, chopped

¼ cup coconut water

1 tsp maple syrup

Preparation:

Combine lettuce and cabbage in a large colander. Rinse under cold running water. Chop into small pieces and set aside.

Peel the papaya and cut lengthwise in half. Scoop out the black seeds and flesh using a spoon. Cut into small chunks and set aside.

Now, combine cabbage, apple, lettuce, and papaya in a juicer. Process until juiced.

Transfer to serving glasses and stir in the coconut water and maple syrup.

Add some ice and serve immediately.

Nutritional information per serving: Kcal: 201, Protein: 7g, Carbs: 61.7g, Fats: 1.7g

28. Broccoli Goji Juice

Ingredients:

1 cup broccoli, pre-cooked

1 cup Goji berries

1 large orange, peeled

1 large cucumber, peeled

2 tsp maple syrup

Preparation:

Wash the broccoli and chop into small pieces. Set aside.

Place the goji berries in a medium bowl. Add 1 cup of water and soak for 30 minutes.

Wash the cucumber and cut into thick slices. Set aside.

Now, combine broccoli, goji berries, and cucumber in a juicer. Process until juiced.

Transfer to serving glasses and stir in the honey.

Add some ice and serve!

Nutritional information per serving: Kcal: 193, Protein: 9.4g, Carbs: 66g, Fats: 1.7g

29.   Vanilla Banana Juice

Ingredients:

1 large banana, sliced

1 large Fuji Apple, cored

1 tsp pure vanilla extract, sugar-free

¼ cup coconut water

Preparation:

Peel the banana and cut into thin slices. Set aside.

Rinse the apple and remove the core. Cut into bite-sized pieces and set aside.

Now, combine banana and apple in a juicer and process until juiced.

Transfer to a serving glass and stir in the vanilla extract and coconut water.

Refrigerate for 10 minutes before serving.

Nutritional information per serving: Kcal: 292, Protein: 6.9g, Carbs: 96g, Fats: 2g

30.   Banana Apple Juice

Ingredients:

1 cup banana, sliced

1 small apple, peeled and seeds removed

1 cup fresh mint leaves, finely chopped

¼ tsp of nutmeg, ground

¼ tsp cinnamon, ground

1 tbsp maple syrup

¼ cup water

Preparation:

Peel the banana and cut into thin slices. Fill the measuring cup and reserve the rest in the refrigerator.

Rinse the apple and remove the core. Cut into bite-sized pieces and set aside.

Now, combine banana, apple and mint in a juicer. Transfer to a serving glasses and stir in the nutmeg, cinnamon, maple syrup, and water

Garnish with some extra mint leaves and refrigerate before serving.

Add some ice and serve immediately.

Nutritional information per serving: Kcal: 141, Protein: 1.5g, Carbs: 41.2g, Fats: 0.4g

31.   Banana Blueberry Juice

Ingredients:

1 large banana, sliced

1 cup blueberries

1 tsp of flaxseeds

½ cup celery, chopped

1 tbsp of honey

Preparation:

Peel the banana and cut into small chunks. Set aside.

Rinse the blueberries under running water. Drain and set aside.

Rinse the celery and chop into bite-sized pieces. Set aside.

Now, combine banana blueberries, and celery in a juicer. Transfer to serving glasses and stir in the flaxseeds and honey.

Add few ice cubes before serving.

Enjoy!

Nutritional information per serving: Kcal: 177, Protein: 6.5g, Carbs: 44.6g, Fats: 2.6g

32.   Kale Strawberry Juice

Ingredients:

1 cup of fresh kale, torn

1 cup of strawberries, fresh

½ tsp of ginger, ground

¼ cup coconut water

Preparation:

Rinse the kale thoroughly under running water. Chop into small pieces and set aside.

Wash the strawberries and remove the stems. Chop into small pieces and set aside.

Combine kale and strawberries in a juicer and process until juiced.

Transfer to serving glasses and stir in the ginger and coconut water. Add some ice cubes before serving.

Enjoy!

Nutritional information per serving: Kcal: 120, Protein: 5.9g, Carbs: 38.6g, Fats: 1.8g

33.   Apple Mango Juice

Ingredients:

1 medium-sized Granny Smith's apple, chopped

1 cup of mango chunks

1 cup of guava chunks

1 tbsp of fresh mint leaves

½ cup of coconut water

Preparation:

Wash the apple and cut in half. Remove the core and cut into bite-sized pieces. Set aside.

Peel the mango and cut into small chunks. Set aside.

Wash the guava and cut into chunks. If you are using large fruit, reserve the rest for some other recipe in a refrigerator.

Now, combine apple, mango, and guava in a juicer. Process until juiced.

Transfer to serving glasses and stir in the coconut water.

Garnish with some mint leaves and add some ice before serving.

Enjoy!

Nutritional information per serving: Kcal: 187, Protein: 3.6g, Carbs: 54.2g, Fats: 1.3g

34.   Carrot Parsnip Juice

Ingredients:

3 large carrots, sliced

1 cup of parsnips, sliced

2 large Fuji apples, peeled and cored

1 tbsp fresh basil, finely chopped

¼ cup of water

Preparation:

Wash the apples and cut into halves. Remove the core and cut into bite-sized pieces. Set aside.

Wash the carrots and parsnips and cut into thick slices. Set aside.

Now, combine carrots, parsnips, and apples in a juicer and process until juiced.

Transfer to serving glasses and stir in the water. Garnish with basil leaves and refrigerate before serving.

Enjoy!

Nutritional information per serving: Kcal: 332, Protein: 5.4g, Carbs: 100g, Fats: 1.6g

35.   Banana Apricot Juice

Ingredients:

1 large banana, sliced

1 cup apricots, chopped

1 large cucumber, sliced

1 cup fresh spinach, torn

½ cup of raw broccoli, chopped

½ cup of pure coconut water

Preparation:

Peel the banana and cut into thin slices. Set aside.

Wash the apricots and cut in half. Remove the pit and chop into chunks. Set aside.

Wash the cucumber and chop into thick slices. Set aside.

Combine spinach and broccoli in a colander and wash under cold running water. Drain and roughly chop. Set aside.

Now, combine banana, apricots, cucumber, spinach, and broccoli in a juicer. Process until juiced. Transfer to serving glasses and stir in the coconut water.

Add some ice and serve immediately.

Nutritional information per serving: Kcal: 218, Protein: 10g, Carbs: 64g, Fats: 1.9g

36.   Mint Cranberry Juice

Ingredients:

1 tbsp fresh mint, finely chopped

1 cup fresh cranberries

2 cups cherries, pitted

1 cup leek, chopped

1 tbsp maple syrup

Preparation:

Wash the cranberries under cold running water and set aside.

Wash the cherries under cold running water. Drain and cut in half. Remove the pits and set aside.

Wash the leek and cut into small pieces. Set aside.

Combine cherries, leek, cranberries, and mint in a juicer and process until juiced.

Transfer to serving glasses and stir in the honey.

Add some ice and serve!

Nutritional information per serving: Kcal: 248, Protein: 5g, Carbs: 75.5g, Fats: 1g

37.   Raspberry Cabbage Juice

Ingredients:

1 cup raspberries

1 cup purple cabbage, torn

1 cup papaya, chopped

1 tsp ginger, ground

1 tsp honey

Preparation:

Rinse the raspberries under cold running water. Drain and set aside.

Rinse the cabbage thoroughly and torn with hands. Set aside.

Peel the papaya and cut lengthwise in half. Scoop out the black seeds and flesh using a spoon. Cut into small chunks and set aside.

Combine raspberries, cabbage, and papaya in a juicer and process until juiced.

Transfer to serving glasses and stir in the ginger and honey.

Add some ice cubes and serve immediately.

Nutritional information per serving: Kcal: 172, Protein: 4.3g, Carbs: 54.2g, Fats: 0.7g

38.   Radish Swiss Chard Juice

Ingredients:

1 large radish, chopped

1 cup Swiss chard, torn

1 large honeydew melon wedge

1 cup asparagus, chopped

1 cup avocado, chopped

¼ cup coconut water

Preparation:

Wash the radish and trim off the green parts. Cut into small pieces and set aside.

Wash the chard thoroughly and torn with hands. Set aside.

Cut the honeydew melon lengthwise in half. Scoop out the seeds using a spoon. Cut the large wedges and peel them. Cut into small chunks and place in a bowl. Wrap the rest of the melon in a plastic foil and refrigerate.

Wash the asparagus and trim off the woody ends. Set aside.

Peel the avocado and cut in half. Remove the pit and cut into chunks. Set aside.

Now, combine radish, chard, melon, asparagus, and avocado in a juicer. Process until juiced.

Transfer to serving glasses and refrigerate 10 minutes before serving.

Nutritional information per serving: Kcal: 275, Protein: 8g, Carbs: 35.2g, Fats: 21.9g

39.   Celery Beet Juice

Ingredients:

1 cup of celery, chopped

1 cup of beets, sliced

1 cup of beet greens, chopped

1 cup of crookneck squash, sliced

1 cup of pomegranate seeds

1 tbsp of honey

Preparation:

Wash the celery and cut into small pieces. Set aside.

Wash the beets and trim off the green parts. Cut into bite-sized pieces and set aside.

Use the trimmed beet greens and roughly chop it.

Wash the crookneck squash and cut in half. Scoop out the seeds using a spoon. Cut into small chunks and set aside. Reserve the rest for another juice.

Cut the top of the pomegranate fruit using a sharp knife. Slice down to each of the white membranes inside of the fruit. Pop the seeds into a measuring cup and set aside.

Now, combine celery, beets, beet greens, celery, and pomegranate seeds in a juicer.

Transfer to serving glasses and stir in the honey.

Add some ice and serve immediately.

Nutritional information per serving: Kcal: 132, Protein: 6.4g, Carbs: 48.8g, Fats: 1.8g

40.   Tomato Swiss Chard Juice

Ingredients:

1 large tomato, chopped

1 cup of Swiss chard, chopped

1 cup of asparagus, trimmed

1 cup of Brussels sprouts, trimmed

1 large cucumber, sliced

Preparation:

Wash the tomato and place in a bowl. Cut into quarters and reserve the juice while cutting. Set aside.

Wash the Swiss chard thoroughly under cold running water. Drain and set aside.

Wash the asparagus and trim off the woody ends. Cut into 1-inch pieces and set aside.

Wash the Brussels sprouts and trim off the outer layers. Cut in half and set aside.

Wash the cucumber and cut into thick slices. Set aside.

Now, combine tomato, Swiss chard, asparagus, Brussels sprouts, and cucumber in a juicer. Process until juiced.

Transfer to serving glasses and add some ice before serving.

Nutrition information per serving: Kcal: 109, Protein: 10.1g, Carbs: 32.4g, Fats: 1.2g

41.   Avocado Cucumber Juice

Ingredients:

1 large tomato, chopped

1 cup avocado, chopped

1 large cucumber, sliced

1 cup of fresh basil, chopped

Preparation:

Peel the avocado and cut in half. Remove the pit and cut into chunks. Fill the measuring cup and reserve the rest for some other juice. Keep it in a refrigerator.

Wash the cucumber and cut into thick slices. Set aside.

Wash the tomato and place in a bowl. Cut into quarters and reserve the juice while cutting. Set aside.

Wash the basil thoroughly and roughly chop it. Set aside.

Now, combine tomato, avocado, cucumber, and basil in a juicer and process until juiced.

Transfer to serving glasses and add some ice before serving.

Enjoy!

Nutrition information per serving: Kcal: 240, Protein: 3.1g, Carbs: 75.1g, Fats: 0.9g

MEALS

Breakfast Recipes

1.   Eggs with Tomato and Spring Onions

Ingredients:

3 whole eggs

1 medium-sized tomato, sliced

3 spring onions, chopped

¼ tsp of salt

¼ tsp of cayenne pepper

2 tbsp of butter

Preparation:

Melt the butter in a frying skillet over a medium-high temperature. Add onions and stir-fry for 2 minutes.

Now add tomato slices, salt and cayenne pepper. Stir-fry tomato slices for about a minute one each side.

Meanwhile, beat the eggs and add to a frying skillet. Cook for about 30 seconds.

Nutrition information per serving: Kcal: 257, Protein: 19g, Carbs: 5g, Fats: 17g

2.   No-Bake Protein Balls with Oats

Ingredients:

1 ½ cup of rolled oats plus

½ cup of peanut butter

¼ cup of minced almonds

3 tablespoons of honey

1 tablespoon of minced chia seeds

1 tbsp of vanilla extract

3 cups of milk

Preparation:

Place one cup of rolled oats in a bowl. Add other dry ingredients and stir to combine.

Now add in peanut butter and honey. Mix well and gently pour in the milk and vanilla extract. Shape the balls using your hands, top with the remaining oats and place in the refrigerator for about 30 minutes.

Nutrition information per serving: Kcal: 425, Protein: 31g, Carbs: 48g, Fats: 10.5g

3.   Chocolate Balls

Ingredients:

1 cup of minced almonds

½ cup of peanut butter

½ cup of honey

2 tablespoons of minced chia seeds

¼ cup of raw cocoa powder

¼ cup of grated dark chocolate

¼ cup of milk

Preparation:

Combine the ingredients in a bowl and mix well to combine. Shape the balls using your hands and refrigerate for about 30 minutes.

Nutrition information per serving: Kcal: 430, Protein: 27g, Carbs: 50g, Fats: 11g

4.   Spinach Omelet

Ingredients:

3 eggs, whole and beaten

½ cup cottage cheese

½ cup of onion, peeled and chopped

1 cup of fresh spinach, finely chopped

1 tbsp of olive oil

salt and pepper, to taste

Preparation:

Heat up the olive oil over a medium temperature. Stir-fry the onions until translucent.

Crack the eggs and mix well with a fork. Add some salt and pepper. Whisk in 1 cup of fresh spinach and ½ cup of cottage cheese. Pour the eggs evenly in a pan and reduce the heat. Cook for about 2 minutes, stirring constantly.

Nutrition information per serving: Kcal: 470, Protein: 32g, Carbs: 9.5g, Fats: 21g

5.   Homemade Fig Spread

Ingredients:

1 pound dry figs, cut into small pieces

6 tbsp powdered stevia

2 tbsp fresh lemon juice

1 cup milk

Preparation:

In a small saucepan, combine the figs, stevia, and fresh lemon juice. Add 1/2 cup of milk and bring it to a boil.

Reduce the heat to low and add the remaining milk. Depending on your taste, you can add some more milk. Cook for about 20 minutes. When done, transfer to a food processor and blend until smooth mixture.

Nutrition information per serving: Kcal: 300, Protein: 5g, Carbs: 66g, Fats: 1g

6.   Pumpkin Seeds Oatmeal

Ingredients:

1 cup of rolled oats

1 tbsp of pumpkin seeds

2 cups of skim milk

½ cup of water

2 egg whites

½ cup of maple syrup

1 tsp of cinnamon, ground

Preparation:

Preheat the oven to 350 degrees. Spread the pumpkin seeds on a baking sheet and toast for about 5-6 minutes. You want a nice lightly brown color.

Boil the 2 cups of skim milk and ½ cup of water over a high temperature. Add the oats, egg whites and stir well. Cook for another 7 minutes, or until the oats are cooked. Stir in the pumpkin seeds. Remove from the heat and let it stand for 10 minutes. Serve with some cinnamon on top.

Nutrition information per serving: Kcal: 168, Protein: 5.1g, Carbs: 30g, Fats: 1.9g

7.   Wild Berries Muesli

Ingredients:

1 cup rolled oats

¼ cup fresh apple juice

½ cup wild berries

2 tbsp honey

1 cup milk

Preparation:

Place the oats in a large bowl. Add fresh apple juice and milk. Cover and let it stand in the refrigerator for about an hour.

Add honey and stir well. Top with wild berries and serve.

Nutrition information per serving: Kcal: 281, Protein: 10g, Carbs: 48g, Fats: 4g

8.   Breakfast Tuna Spread

Ingredients:

1 medium-sized tuna fillet

1 small onion, peeled

3 tbsp olive oil

¼ tsp black pepper

¼ tsp sea salt

1 tsp dry rosemary

Preparation:

Wash and pat dry the fillet. Cut into bite size pieces and set aside.

Heat up the oil in a large skillet and add the tuna chops. Cook for about ten minutes stirring constantly. Remove from the heat.

Meanwhile, combine the ingredients in a blender. Add tuna and mix well for about 30 seconds. Enjoy!

Nutrition information per serving: Kcal: 275, Protein: 26g, Carbs: 0g, Fats: 19g

9.   Grilled Eggplant Slices

Ingredients:

1 large eggplant

3 eggs

¼ tsp of sea salt

1 tbsp of olive oil

½ tsp of cinnamon

Preparation:

Peel eggplant and cut into slices. Sprinkle some salt on each side of eggplant. Allow it to rest for about 15 minutes. Meanwhile, mix eggs with cinnamon in a large bowl. Heat up the olive oil in frying pan over a medium temperature.

Put the eggplant slices in the egg mixture. Make few holes with a knife to allow the mixture to permeate the eggplant. Fry it until golden brown color, on each side. This should take about 10 minutes. Serve your eggplant slices warm.

Nutrition information per serving: Kcal: 65, Protein: 3.8g, Carbs: 9g, Fats: 3.6g

10.   Scrambled Eggs with Turmeric

Ingredients:

2 eggs

1 egg white

1 tbsp of olive oil

1 tsp of ground turmeric

salt and pepper to taste

Preparation:

Grease the frying pan with olive oil. Heat up over to medium-high heat. Meanwhile, whisk together eggs, egg white and turmeric. Add some salt and pepper to taste and fry for few minutes.

Nutrition information per serving: Kcal: 71, Protein: 21g, Carbs: 2g, Fats: 8g

Lunch Recipes

11.   Tortellini with Cheese Sauce

Ingredients:

1 (16 ounces) package frozen cheese tortellini (choose rice flour, vegan tortellini)

3 cups of vegetable broth

1 cup of cashew cream

2 tbsp of whipped cooking cream, dairy-free

2oz tofu, grated

¼ tsp of cayenne pepper

A handful of fresh parsley, finely chopped

Preparation:

In a deep pot, bring 3 cups of vegetable broth to boil. Add frozen cheese tortellini and cook for 3-4 minutes. (The cooking time depends on your tortellini. Use package instructions). Remove from the heat and drain.

Reduce the heat to minimum and add the grated tofu. Slowly pour in the cashew cream, whipped cooking cream and cayenne pepper. Cook for a couple of minutes.

Transfer the tortellini to a plate, top with cheese sauce and sprinkle with chopped parsley.

Serve warm.

Nutrition information per 1 serving: Kcal: 521 Protein: 28g, Carbs: 56.4g, Fats: 13g

12.   Pressure Cooker's Beans

Ingredients:

1 ½ pound of beans, pre - cooked

2 medium – sized carrots, sliced

1 large red pepper, chopped

2 medium – sized onions, sliced

5 gloves of garlic, minced

3 small – sized tomatoes, sliced

1 cup of tomato sauce

1 small chili pepper

1 cup of sliced celery

2 tbsp of olive oil

7 glasses of water

Preparation:

With the cooker's lid off, heat the olive oil on high. Stir-fry the onions for 2 minutes.

Add sliced carrots, pepper and garlic. Cook for about 10 minutes on high temperature. Then add the tomatoes, tomato sauce, and 1 more glass of hot water.

Add the pre-cooked beans and 5 glasses of water. Now add the celery and chili pepper.

Securely lock the cooker's lid. Set for 10 minutes on high.

Nutrition information per 1 serving: Kcal: 356 Protein: 9g, Carbs: 49g, Fats: 6g

13.   Roasted Chicken

Ingredients:

1 whole chicken

1 tsp salt

Preparation:

Wash and clean the chicken. Evenly sprinkle the salt all over chicken.

Preheat the oven to 350 degrees F. Place the chicken in a baking sheet, over a baking paper.

Roast for about an hour.

Nutrition information per 1 serving: Kcal: 371 Protein: 38g, Carbs: 0g, Fats: 16g

14.   Moroccan Rice

Ingredients:

1 cup of brown rice

2 tbsp. extra virgin olive oil

2 medium-sized carrots, grated

1 small tomato, peeled and finely chopped

1 tbsp. Moroccan spice seasoning

1 medium-sized onion, peeled and chopped

6-7 dried apricots, halved

Preparation:

In a deep pot, bring 3 cups of water to a boiling point. Add rice, reduce the heat to minimum, and cook until the water evaporates. Remove from the heat.

Heat up the olive oil in a frying pan. Add onion and stir-fry until translucent. Now add tomato, apricots, and Moroccan spice seasoning. Cook for five more minutes and add rice. Stir well to combine.

Top with grated carrots and serve.

Nutrition information per 1 serving: Kcal: 435 Protein: 15.9g, Carbs: 67g, Fats: 6.3g

15.   Broccoli Stew

Ingredients:

2oz fresh broccoli

A handful of fresh parsley, finely chopped

1 tsp of dry thyme

1 tbsp of fresh lemon juice

¼ tsp of ground chili pepper

3 tbsp of olive oil

1 tbsp of cashew cream

Preparation:

Place the broccoli in a deep pot and pour enough water to cover. Bring it to a boil and cook until tender. Remove from the heat and drain.

Transfer to a food processor. Add fresh parsley, thyme, and about ½ cup of water. Pulse until smooth mixture. Return to a pot and add some more water. Bring it to a boil and cook for several minutes, over a minimum temperature.

Stir in some olive oil and cashew cream, sprinkle with ground chili pepper and add fresh lemon juice. Serve warm.

Nutrition information per 1 serving: Kcal: 72 Protein: 12g, Carbs: 15.8g, Fats: 8g

16.   Light Mac and Tuna

Ingredients:

1 cup of minced tuna

½ cup of homemade cashew cream

2 cups of rice flour macaroni

1 tsp of sea salt

1 tsp of olive oil

1 tbsp of canola oil

Few olives for decoration (optional)

Preparation:

Pour 3 cups of water in a pot. Bring it to boil and add macaroni and salt. Boil macaroni for about 3 minutes (rice flour macaroni take less time to cook). You can also use the package instructions to cook macaroni, if you're not sure. Remove from heat and drain.

In a bowl, combine tuna with homemade cashew cream. Mash well with a fork.

In a large saucepan, combine the olive oil with canola oil. Heat up over a medium temperature and add tuna mixture. Fry for about 15-20 minutes stirring occasionally. Add macaroni and mix well. Cover the saucepan and allow macaroni to heat up. Serve warm with some olives.

Nutrition information per serving: Kcal: 224, Protein: 33g, Carbs: 44.3g, Fats: 12g

17.   Orange Barbecue Chicken

Ingredients:

2 pounds of chicken tighs

2 medium onions, chopped

2 small chili peppers

1 cup of chicken broth

¼ cup of fresh orange juice

1 tsp of orange extract

2 tbsp of olive oil

1 tsp of barbecue seasoning mix

1 small red onion, chopped

Preparation:

Heat up the olive oil in a large saucepan. Add chopped onions and fry for several minutes, over a medium temperature – until golden color.

Combine chili peppers, orange juice and orange extract. Mix well in a food processor for 20-30 seconds. Add this mixture into a saucepan and stir well. Reduce heat to simmer.

Coat the chicken with barbecue seasoning mix and put into a saucepan. Add chicken broth and bring it to a boil. Cook over a medium temperature until the water evaporates. Remove from the heat.

Preheat the oven to 350 degrees. Place the chicken into a large baking dish. Bake for about 15 minutes to get a nice crispy, golden brown color.

Nutrition information per serving: Kcal: 170 Protein: 38g, Carbs: 11g, Fats: 21g

18. Grilled Veal Steak with Vegetables

Ingredients:

1 pound of veal steak, about 1 inch thick

1 medium red pepper

1 medium green pepper

1 small onion

3 tbsp of olive oil

Salt and pepper to taste

Preparation:

Wash and pat dry the steak with a kitchen paper. Heat up the olive oil over a medium temperature and fry the meat for about 20 minutes (about 10 on each side). Remove from the heat and set aside.

Wash and cut vegetables into thin strips. Add some salt and pepper. Cook for about 15 minutes stirring constantly.

Serve immediately.

Nutrition information per serving: Calories: 309 Protein: 35g Carbohydrates: 7.1g Fats: 17g

19.   Easy Chicken Stew

Ingredients:

1 pound of chicken thighs

3 cups of chicken broth

3 red onions, chopped

2 large carrots, chopped

2 medium-sized sweet potatoes

½ tsp of salt

¼ tsp of peper

Preparation:

Place the ingredients in a deep pot. Add chicken broth and season with salt and pepper.

Set the heat to minimum and cook for about two hours, or until the meat is done and vegetables soft.

Nutrition information per serving: Calories490 Protein: 62g Carbohydrates: 39g Fats: 23g

20.   Pan Roasted Lamb with Rice

Ingredients:

2 pounds of lamb cutlets, boneless

1 cup of brown rice

2 ½ cup of water

1 tsp of ground turmeric

5 tbsp of olive oil

¼ cup of lemon juice

3 cloves of garlic, minced

½ tsp of sea salt

½ tsp of ground pepper

1 tbsp of rice flour

¼ cup of water

Preparation:

Boil 2 ½ cup of water and add rice. Cook over medium temperature for about 10 minutes, or until the water evaporates. Remove from the heat and add ground turmeric. This will give your rice a nice golden color but it will also add some amazing nutritional values to your food. Cover the rice and set aside.

Wash and pat dry the cutlets. Heat up the olive oil over a medium temperature. Add the cutlets into a skillet and cook for about 10 minutes on each side. Reduce the heat to low and add rice flour, minced garlic, lemon juice, salt, pepper and some more water (¼ cup should be enough). Stir well and cook for about 15 minutes.

Serve with rice.

Nutrition information per serving: Calories: 411 Protein: 45g Carbohydrates: 19g Fats: 21g

Dinner Recipes:

21.   Marinated Salmon Slices

Ingredients:

2 pounds of fresh salmon, sliced into 1 inch slices

1 cup of extra virgin olive oil

3 tbsp of freshly squeezed lemon juice

1 tbsp of finely chopped rosemary

1 tsp of dry oregano, ground

1 dry bay leaf, crushed

1 tsp of salt

1 tbsp of cayenne pepper

Preparation:

Combine the olive oil with lemon juice, chopped rosemary, dry oregano, bay leaf, salt, and cayenne pepper. Stir well to combine.

Using a kitchen brush, spread this mixture over the salmon sliced. Let it stand for about 10-15 minutes.

Meanwhile, preheat the grill pan over a medium-high heat. Grill the salmon slices for 3 minutes, on each side.

Nutrition information per serving: Calories: 261 Protein: 26g Carbohydrates: 0g Fats: 16g

22.   Citrus Sea Bream

Ingredients:

1 piece of fresh sea bream

1 cup of olive oil

½ lemon, sliced

¼ cup of freshly squeezed lemon juice

1 tsp of dry rosemary, ground

1 tbsp of fresh parsley, finely chopped

3 garlic cloves, crushed

¼ tsp of sea salt

Preparation:

Wash and clean the fish. Pat dry and cut in half.

Combine the olive oil, lemon juice, dry rosemary, fresh parsley, crushed garlic cloves, and sea salt in a large bowl. Soak the fish in this marinate and leave in the refrigerator for at least 30 minutes (it can stand in the refrigerator up to 2 hours).

Meanwhile, preheat the oven to 300 degrees. Spread some olive oil over a baking sheet and set aside.

Remove the fish from the refrigerator and transfer to a baking sheet. Add some of the marinade and cook for about 30 minutes.

Remove from the oven, sprinkle with some more marinade and serve with lemon slices and some vegetables of your choice.

Nutrition information per serving: Calories: 175 Protein: 31g Carbohydrates: 0.5g Fats: 21g

23.   Vegetable Risotto

Ingredients:

1 cup of brown rice

1 medium-sized carrot, sliced

1 medium-sized zucchini, sliced

1 small tomato, roughly chopped

½ small eggplant, sliced

1 small red pepper, sliced

3 tbsp of extra virgin olive oil

½ tsp of salt

1 tsp of dry marjoram

Preparation:

Place the rice in a deep pot. Add 2 cups of water and bring it to a boil. Reduce the heat and cook until the water evaporates. Stir occasionally.

Heat up one tablespoon of olive oil over a medium-high heat. Add sliced carrot and stir-fry for 3-4 minutes, stirring constantly. Combine with rice.

Stir in the remaining olive oil, zucchini, tomato, eggplant, red pepper, salt, and marjoram. Add one cup of water and continue to cook for another 10 minutes.

Nutrition information per serving: Calories: 220 Protein: 6g Carbohydrates: 51g Fats: 7.8g

24.   Grilled Broccoli

Ingredients:

4oz fresh broccoli

Freshly ground black pepper to taste

Fresh parsley, chopped

3 tbsp of olive oil

Preparation:

Heat up the olive oil in a large grill pan. Place the broccoli and grill for 5-6 minutes, or until lightly charred.

Transfer to a plate and sprinkle with some pepper and parsley. Serve warm.

Serving tip:

Combine the chopped parsley with one garlic clove.

Nutrition information per 1 serving: Kcal: 40 Protein: 3.2g, Carbs: 7.5g, Fats: 3g

25.   Grilled Trout

Ingredients:

7oz fresh trout steaks

¼ cup of chopped fresh coriander leaves

2 garlic cloves, minced

¼ cup of tablespoons of lemon juice

½ teaspoon smoked paprika

½ teaspoon cumin, ground

½ teaspoon chili powder

Ground black pepper to taste

Preparation:

Add the coriander, crushed garlic, paprika, cumin, chili powder, and lemon juice in a food processor and pulse to combine.

Transfer the mixture into a bowl, add the fish and gently toss to coat the fish evenly with sauce. Chill for at least 2 hours to allow the flavor to penetrate into the fish.

Remove the fish from the refrigerator and preheat the grill pan. Place the fish and grill for about 3 to 4 minutes on each side.

Remove the fish from the grill, transfer on a serving plate and serve with lemon or some vegetables of your choice.

Nutrition information per 1 serving: Kcal: 143 Protein: 21g, Carbs: 0g, Fats: 7g

26.   Grilled zucchini

Ingredients:

4oz zucchini

¼ cup of fresh lemon juice

¼ tsp of sea salt

1 tsp dry rosemary

¼ tsp of freshly ground black pepper

Preparation:

Whisk together lemon juice, sea salt, rosemary, and black pepper. Wash and peel zucchini. Cut into thin slices. Brush each slice with this mixture.

Preheat a non-stick grill pan, or an electric grill, over a medium-high temperature. Grill the zucchini for several minutes on each side. Serve warm.

Nutrition information per 1 serving: Kcal: 18 Protein: 1.3g, Carbs: 3.8g, Fats: 0.2g

27.   Grilled Shrimps

Ingredients:

2 lbs fresh large shrimps, whole

3 tbsp. extra-virgin olive oil

Sea salt to taste

Preparation:

Make sure you use the best, extra-virgin olive oil for to get a maximum flavor.

Heat up some olive oil in a grill pan, over a medium-high heat. Three tablespoons will be enough. Place the shrimps in it and grill for 5 minutes, turning to char all sides.

Remove from the heat and use some kitchen paper to soak up the excess oil.

Transfer to a plate and sprinkle with some salt. Serve immediately.

Nutrition information per serving: Kcal: 224, Protein: 27.1g, Carbs: 10g, Fats: 5g

Add extra flavor:

Extra virgin olive oil is definitely one of my favorite ingredients in food. Its tender flavor and a unique smell is not the only reason why this liquid gold is so popular. Olive oil is loaded with antioxidants and healthy fats. Its health benefits are something everybody agrees on. A drizzle of olive oil in this protein-packed meal will protect your heart and blood vessels. And to make things even more interesting, healthy garlic and chopped parsley topping will turn the shrimps into a poetry of flavors.

In a small bowl, combine 1 cup of olive oil with 1 tbsp. of finely chopped parsley, 2 crushed garlic cloves, 1 tsp of dry rosemary, ½ tsp of salt, ¼ tsp of pepper. Use to marinate the shrimps before grilling.

Drizzle two tablespoons of this marinade over grilled shrimps. Tastes perfect every time!

28. Stewed Spinach

Ingredients:

7oz fresh spinach

2 tbsp fresh coriander, finely chopped

1 tsp apple cider vinegar

3 tbsp extra virgin olive oil

Fresh water

Preparation:

Fill in a large saucepan with fresh water and bring to a boil. Wash the spinach and add to the saucepan. Cover and reduce the heat to minimum. Cook for about 2-3 minutes, until spinach has wilted.

Remove from the heat and drain. Allow it to cool for a while.

Transfer the spinach to a skillet. Add olive oil and stir-fry for several minutes, stirring constantly. Remove from the heat and season with fresh coriander and apple cider vinegar.

Nutrition information per serving: Kcal: 38, Protein: 3g, Carbs: 5g, Fats: 7g

29. Lettuce Wraps

Ingredients:

1 pound of salmon meat, minced

1 tablespoon mixed vegetable seasoning

¼ cup minced red onion

2 tablespoons bell pepper, minced

½ cup tomato puree

8 large Iceberg lettuce leaves

½ cup cashew cream

Olive oil

½ cup of water or chicken stock

Preparation:

Heat up some oil in a non-stick pan over medium-high temperature. Add the salmon meat and cook for 5 minutes, stirring constantly. Stir in the vegetable seasoning, onions, bell pepper and tomato puree and cook it for 5 minutes. Pour in the water or stock, cover with lid and bring it to a boil. Reduce the heat to low and simmer for about 20 minutes, or until the liquid has reduced in half. Remove the pan from heat and set it aside.

Prepare the lettuce leaves and place them on a work surface. Portion the meat into the 6 to 8 lettuce leaves. Add cashew cream and wrap.

Nutrition information per serving: Kcal: 249, Protein: 20.5g, Carbs: 7g, Fats: 16g

30.   Grilled Tuna Steaks

Ingredients:

¼ cup of chopped fresh coriander leaves

3 garlic cloves, minced

2 tablespoons of lemon juice

½ cup olive oil

4 tuna steaks

½ teaspoon smoked paprika

½ teaspoon cumin, ground

½ teaspoon chili powder

Salt and black pepper

Preparation:

Add the coriander, garlic, paprika, cumin, chili powder and lemon juice in a food processor and pulse to combine. Gradually add in the oil and mix the ingredients until a smooth mixture.

Transfer the mixture into a bowl, add the fish and gently toss to coat the fish evenly with sauce. Chill for at least 2 hours to allow the flavors to penetrate into the fish.

Remove the fish from the chiller and preheat the grill. Lightly brush the grid with oil, place the fish and grill for about 3 to 4 minutes on each side.

Remove the fish from the grill, transfer on a serving plate and serve with lemon wedges or some vegetables

Nutrition information per serving: Kcal: 110, Protein: 25g, Carbs: 0g, Fats: 4g

Salad Recipes

31.   Cucumber Salad

Ingredients:

3.5 oz cucumber, peeled and sliced

1 tbsp of fresh lime juice

3 tbsp of extra virgin olive oil

2 tbsp of finely chopped parsley

2 garlic cloves

½ tsp of salt

¼ tsp of freshly ground black pepper

Preparation:

Peel and slice the cucumber. Transfer to a serving platter. Combine the olive oil with fresh lime juice, chopped parsley, crushed garlic cloves, salt, and pepper. Stir well to combine. Pour the mixture over cucumber and let it stand in the refrigerator for about one hour before serving.

Nutrition information per serving: Kcal: 121, Protein: 2g, Carbs: 3g, Fats: 13g

32.   Rice Salad

Ingredients:

1 cup of long grain, brown rice

3 spring onions, finely chopped

½ cup of sweet corn

1 medium-sized red bell pepper

A handful of chopped mint

2 tbsp of extra virgin olive oil

1 tbsp of apple cider vinegar

Salt to taste

Preparation:

Place the rice in a deep pot. Add 3 cups of water and bring it to a boil. Reduce the heat, cover and simmer until the water evaporates. Remove from the heat and cool.

Combine the ingredients in a deep bowl. Add olive oil, apple cider vinegar, and some salt to taste. Toss well to combine.

Serve cold.

Nutrition information per serving: Kcal: 395 Protein: 2g, Carbs: 38g, Fats: 18g

33. Fresh Vegetable Salad

Ingredients:

3.5oz lettuce, roughly chopped

1 onion, peeled and sliced

1 medium-sized tomato, chopped

A handful of soy beans, soaked

3 tbsp of extra virgin olive oil

1 tbsp of apple cider vinegar

1 tsp of fresh rosemary, finely chopped

¼ tsp of salt

Preparation:

In a small bowl combine the olive oil with apple cider vinegar, rosemary, and salt. Mix well to combine.

Place the vegetables in a large bowl. Add soaked soy beans and drizzle with marinade.

Serve cold.

Nutrition information per serving: Kcal: 145 Protein: 19g, Carbs: 14g, Fats: 11g

34.   Sweet Carrot Salad

Ingredients:

1 medium-sized carrot, sliced

2oz baby spinach

1 medium-sized tomato, finely chopped

2oz rice spaghetti, soaked

1 small tomato, finely chopped

¼ cup of fresh blueberries

For the dressing:

¼ cup of honey

¼ cup of fresh lime juice

1 tsp of dijon mustard

¼ tbsp of ground cumin

Preparation:

Soak the rice spaghetti in water for about 15 minutes. Drain and transfer to a bowl.

Add chopped spinach, tomato, sliced carrot, and blueberries. Toss to combine.

In another bowl, combine the marinade ingredients and mix well. Drizzle over salad.

Serve.

Nutrition information per serving: Kcal: 98 Protein: 4.5g, Carbs: 19g, Fats: 6g

35.   Spring Salad with Black Olives

Ingredients:

5 cherry tomatoes, whole

A handful of black olives

1 medium-sized onion, peeled and sliced

2 radishes, sliced

A handful of lamb's lettuce

2 tbsp of freshly squeezed lime juice

3 tbsp of extra virgin olive oil

Salt to taste

Preparation:

Place the vegetables in a large bowl. Add olive oil, fresh lime juice and some salt to taste. Toss to combine.

Nutrition information per serving: Kcal: 41 Protein: 1g, Carbs: 7g, Fats: 4g

36.   Green Bean Salad

Ingredients:

1 pound green beans

¼ cup of extra virgin olive oil

2 garlic cloves, crushed

1 tbsp of lime juice

Preparation:

Boil a pot of water and add one teaspoon of salt and green beans. Cook until tender. Rinse and drain.

Meanwhile, combine the crushed garlic with olive oil and lime juice. Pour over beans and serve.

Nutrition information per serving: Kcal: 138 Protein: 5g, Carbs: 18g, Fats: 6.7g

37. Raspberry Salad

Ingredients:

A handful of lettuce, torn

1 tbsp of pumpkin seeds

1 cup of fresh raspberries

1 tbsp of fresh rosemary, chopped

2 tbsp of fresh lime juice

1 tsp of cumin

1 tsp of agave syrup

Preparation:

Combine the lettuce with pumpkin seeds and raspberries in a bowl. In a separate bowl, combine the agave syrup with lime juice, cumin, and fresh rosemary. Drizzle over salad and serve.

Nutrition information per serving: Kcal: 29 Protein: 4g, Carbs: 10g, Fats: 3g

38.   Cherry Tomatoes with Broccoli

Ingredients

2 cups of broccoli, cut in half

2 large tomatoes, chopped roughly

2 tbsp of olive oil

1 tbsp of dry salad seasoning of your choice (I use dry parsley)

salt to taste

3 cups of water

Preparation:

Bring the water to boil in a deep pot. Add broccoli and cook for about 20 minutes, or until soft. You can try this with a fork. Remove from the heat and drain. Allow it to cool for a while and cut each broccoli in half. Wash and roughly chop the tomatoes. Combine it with broccoli in a bowl and season with olive oil and salad seasoning.

You can add a few garlic cloves, but this is optional.

Nutrition information per serving: Kcal: 88 Protein: 7g, Carbs: 31g, Fats: 12g

39.   Seafood Salad

Ingredients:

1 small pack of frozen mixed seafood

1 tbsp of olive oil

1 small onion

1 cup of cherry tomatoes

1 tsp of chopped, dry rosemary

1 tbsp of sweet corn

¼ tsp of salt

1 tbsp of freshly squeezed lemon juice

Preparation

Heat up the olive oil in a saucepan. Fry frozen seafood for about 15 minutes, over a medium temperature (try the octopus, it takes the most time to tender). You can add some water if necessary – about ¼ of cup will be enough. Stir occasionally. Remove from frying pan and allow it to cool for about an hour.

Meanwhile, chop the vegetables into very small pieces. In a large bowl, combine the vegetables with corn, seafood and season with salt, rosemary and lemon juice.

Nutrition information per serving: Kcal: 315 Protein: 27g, Carbs: 15g, Fats: 12g

40.   Dandelion Greens Salad

Ingredients:

2oz fresh dandelion greens, roughly chopped

1oz tomato, finely chopped

½ cup of fresh lemon juice

1 tbsp of mustard

Sea salt to taste

Preparation:

Roughly chop the dandelion greens and place in a bowl. Pour the lemon juice over it and let it stand for about 30 minutes. Remove from the bowl and drain. Add finely chopped tomato and mustard. Season with salt and one teaspoon of apple cider vinegar. Serve immediately.

Nutrition information per serving: Kcal: 31 Protein: 2.3g, Carbs: 7.1g, Fats: 0.5g

Snack Recipes

41.   Green Bean Puree

Ingredients:

4oz fresh green beans

Spices of your choice

Preparation:

Clean the beans and place in a pot. Add enough water and cook until tender. Remove from the heat and rinse well under the cold water. Place in a food processor and mix until smooth mixture. Season with some spices of your choice and serve warm.

Nutrition information per serving: Kcal: 35 Protein: 2.5g, Carbs: 8g, Fats: 0.3g

42.   Broccoli Soup

Ingredients:

2oz fresh broccoli

A handful of fresh parsley, finely chopped

1 tsp of dry thyme

1 tbsp of fresh lemon juice

¼ tsp of ground chili pepper

Preparation:

Place the broccoli in a deep pot and pour enough water to cover. Bring it to a boil and cook until tender. Remove from the heat and drain. Transfer to a food processor. Add fresh parsley, thyme, and about ½ cup of water. Pulse until smooth mixture. Return to a pot and add some more water. Bring it to a boil and cook for several minutes, over a minimum temperature. Sprinkle with ground chili pepper and add fresh lemon juice. Serve warm.

Nutrition information per serving: Kcal: 19 Protein: 1.6g, Carbs: 3.7g, Fats: 0.2g

43.   Mashed broccoli with Mint

Ingredients:

8oz broccoli, chopped

1 cup of coconut milk

1 tbsp of vanilla extract

1 tsp of dry mint (or any other seasoning of your choice)

Preparation:

Place the broccoli in a deep pot. Add enough water to cover. Bring it to a boil and cook for 15-20 minutes, or until soft. When done, drain and drain and transfer to a food processor. Add dry mint, coconut milk, and vanilla extract. Pulse to combine. If the mixture is too thick, you can add some more coconut milk.

Nutrition information per serving: Kcal: 32 Protein: 17g, Carbs: 8g, Fats: 5g

ADDITIONAL TITLES FROM THIS AUTHOR

70 Effective Meal Recipes to Prevent and Solve Being Overweight: Burn Fat Fast by Using Proper Dieting and Smart Nutrition

By

Joe Correa CSN

48 Acne Solving Meal Recipes: The Fast and Natural Path to Fixing Your Acne Problems in Less Than 10 Days!

By

Joe Correa CSN

41 Alzheimer's Preventing Meal Recipes: Reduce or Eliminate Your Alzheimer's Condition in 30 Days or Less!

By

Joe Correa CSN

70 Effective Breast Cancer Meal Recipes: Prevent and Fight Breast Cancer with Smart Nutrition and Powerful Foods

By

Joe Correa CSN

www.ingramcontent.com/pod-product-compliance
Lightning Source LLC
Chambersburg PA
CBHW030252030426
42336CB00009B/359